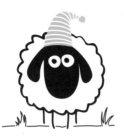

THIS BOOK WILL MAKE YOU FALL ASLEEP

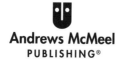

Andrews McMeel
PUBLISHING®

Andrews McMeel Publishing
A division of Andrews McMeel Universal
1130 Walnut Street, Kansas City, Missouri 64106

www.andrewsmcmeel.com

First published in 2019 by Summersdale Publishers Ltd.
Part of Octopus Publishing Group Limited
Carmelite House, 50 Victoria Embankment
London, EC4Y 0DZ, UK

19 20 21 22 23 SHO 10 9 8 7 6 5 4 3 2 1

ISBN: 978-1-5248-5530-7

Library of Congress Control Number: 2019944768

Editor: Jean Z. Lucas
Art Director: Holly Swayne
Production Manager: Tamara Haus
Production Editor: Margaret Daniels

Attention: Schools and Businesses
Andrews McMeel books are available at quantity discounts
with bulk purchase for educational, business, or sales
promotional use. For information, please e-mail the
Andrews McMeel Publishing Special Sales Department:
specialsales@amuniversal.com.

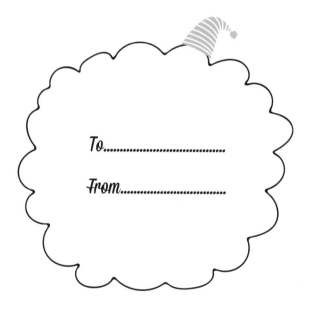

To.....................................

From..................................

INTRODUCTION

Are you tired of sleepless nights? Do you wish you could drop off in two shakes of lamb's tail? Then say hello to Kip!

Follow your new woolly friend through this book. Complete the puzzles and count the sheep when they appear, feel your eyes grow heavier with each turn of the page, and allow Kip to guide you through to the Land of Nod. You will be snoozing in no time!

Find answers to the puzzles on pages 158-9

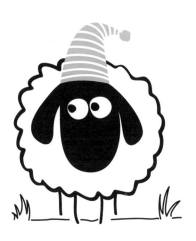

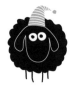

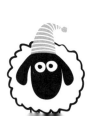

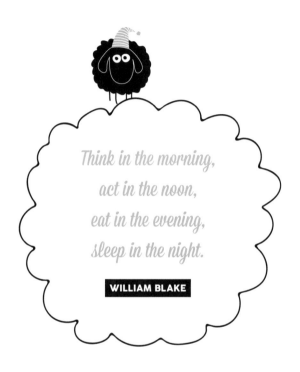

Think in the morning,
act in the noon,
eat in the evening,
sleep in the night.

WILLIAM BLAKE

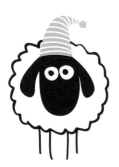

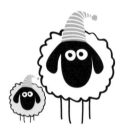

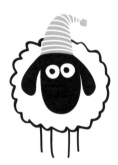

GUIDE KIP
TO THE PILLOW

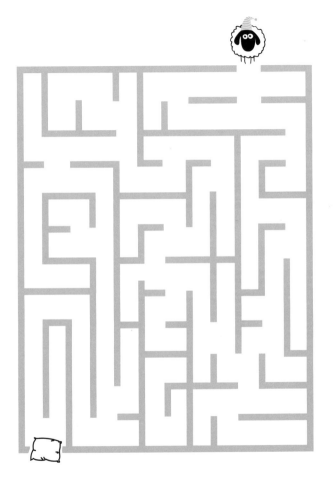

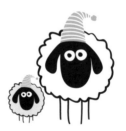
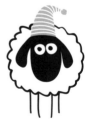

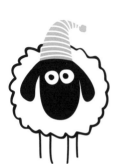

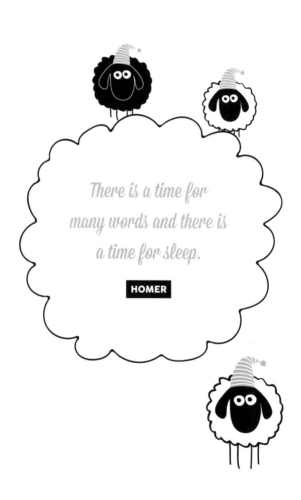

There is a time for
many words and there is
a time for sleep.

HOMER

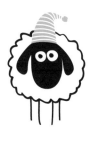
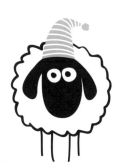

GUIDE KIP TO THE PILLOW

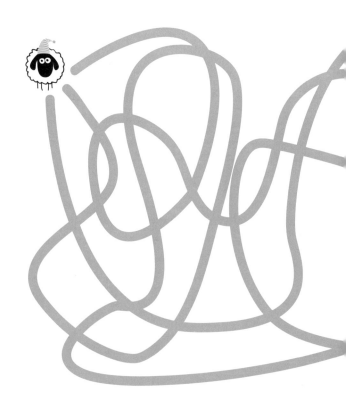

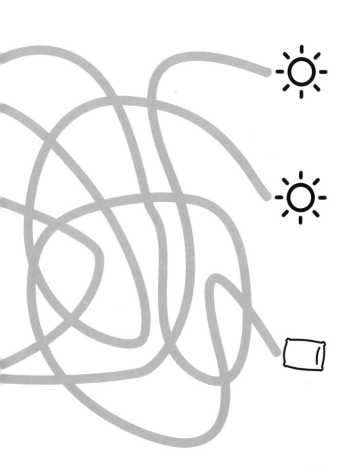

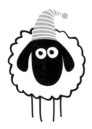

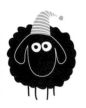
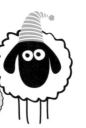
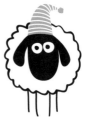

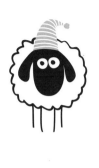
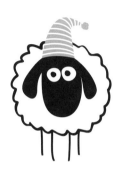

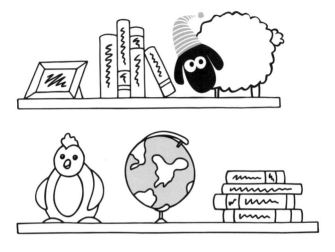

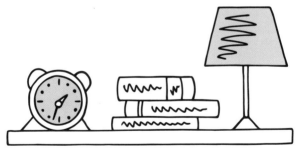

Make your bedroom a sanctuary so that you'll look forward to bedtime. Keep it clean and tidy, use soft lighting, and only have pictures and trinkets that bring you joy.

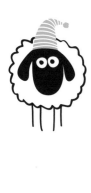
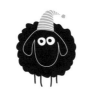

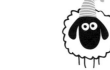
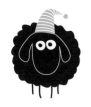

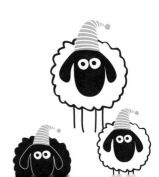

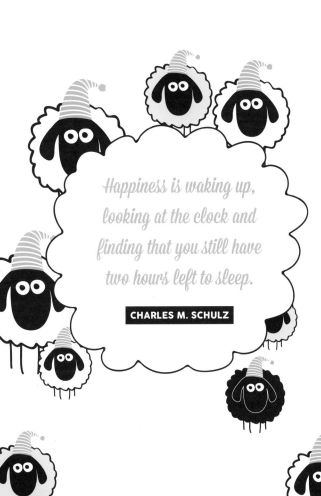

Happiness is waking up,
looking at the clock and
finding that you still have
two hours left to sleep.

CHARLES M. SCHULZ

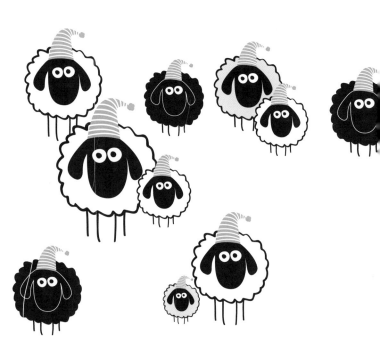
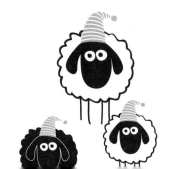

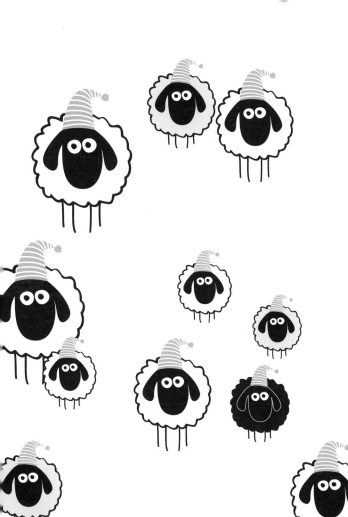

COMPLETE THE WORD SEARCH

dream

doze

nap

rest

snooze

t	p	c	a	d	r	n	i
e	d	r	e	a	m	p	q
c	o	n	x	m	u	a	k
e	z	o	o	n	s	p	y
f	e	t	p	j	l	w	n
a	w	q	s	m	o	r	p
r	l	n	c	e	t	x	a
o	v	e	p	w	r	m	n

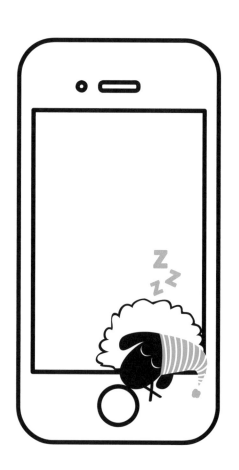

SWITCH OFF YOUR GADGETS
AT LEAST HALF AN HOUR BEFORE
BEDTIME TO ALLOW YOUR
MIND TO WIND
DOWN AND PREPARE
ITSELF FOR SLEEP.

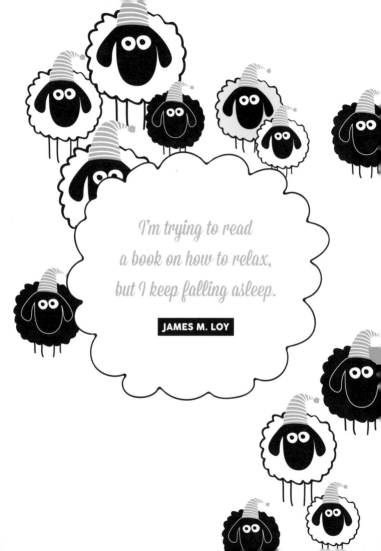

I'm trying to read
a book on how to relax,
but I keep falling asleep.

JAMES M. LOY

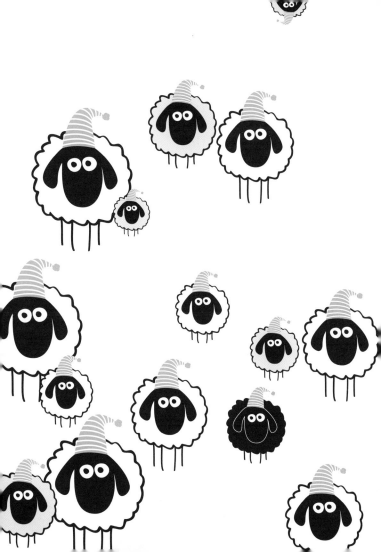

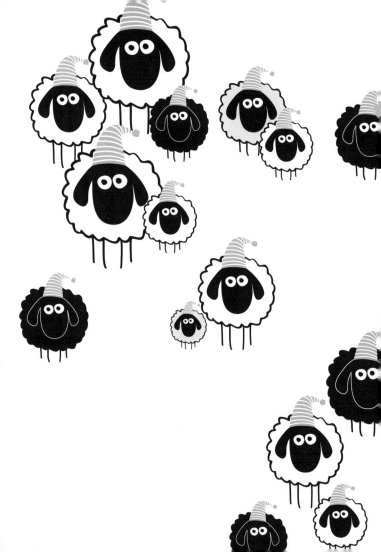

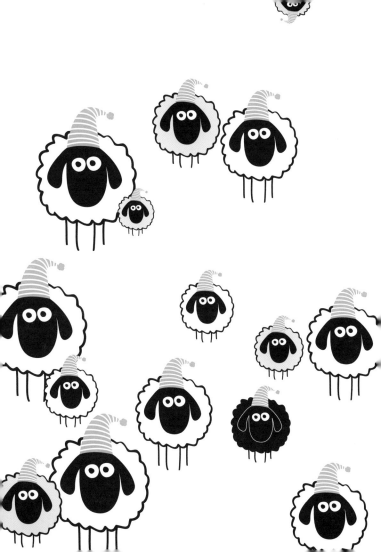

Spot the five differences

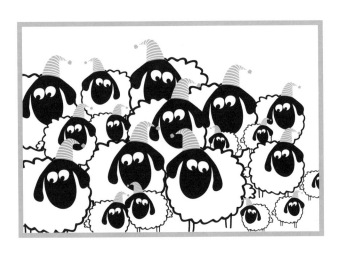

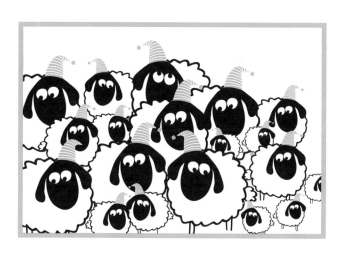

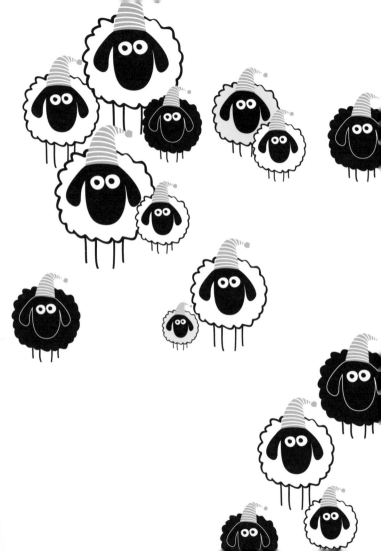

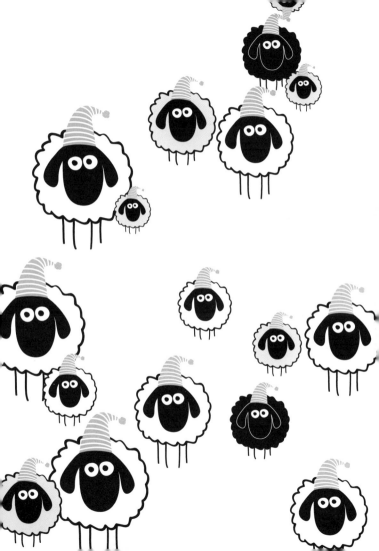

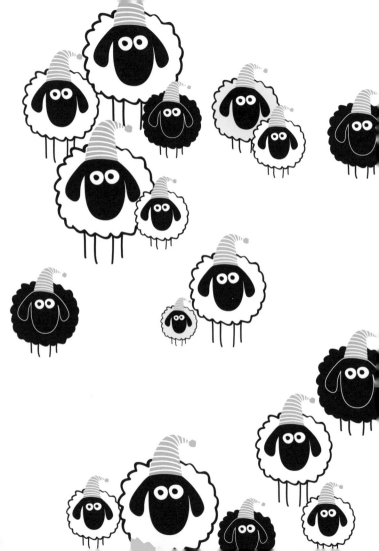

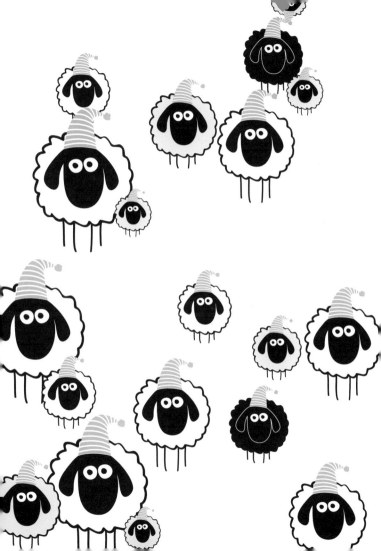

Guide Kip
to the pillow

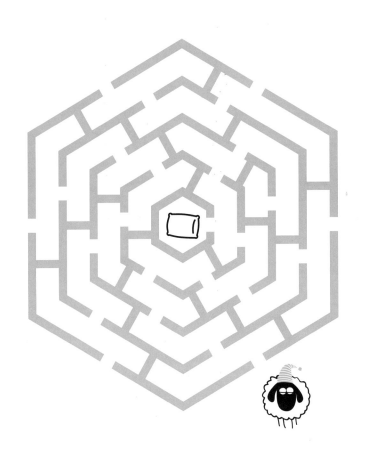

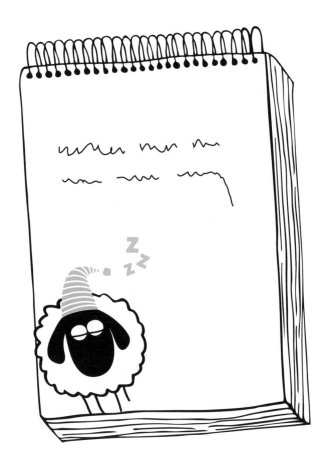

Write in a journal before you go to sleep. Getting your worries out of your head and onto paper can help clear your mind and make you feel calm.

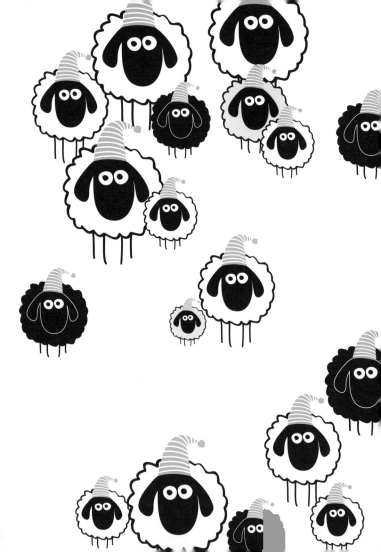

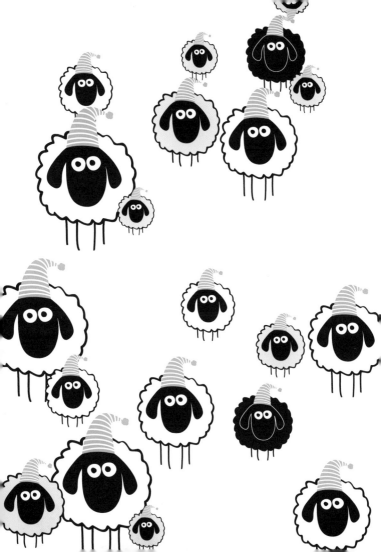

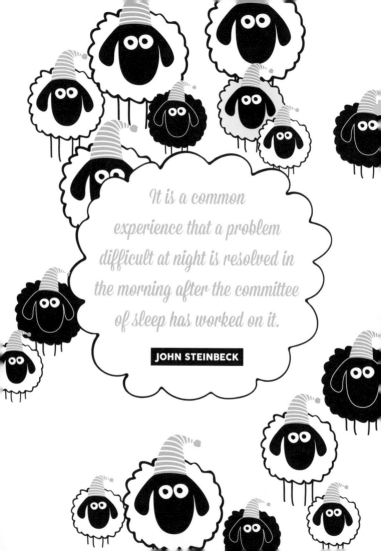

It is a common experience that a problem difficult at night is resolved in the morning after the committee of sleep has worked on it.

JOHN STEINBECK

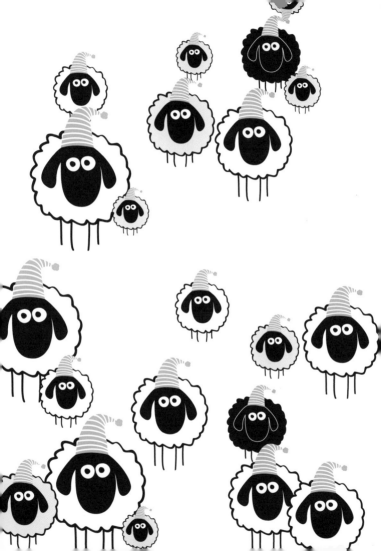

FIND THE SLEEPING SHEEP

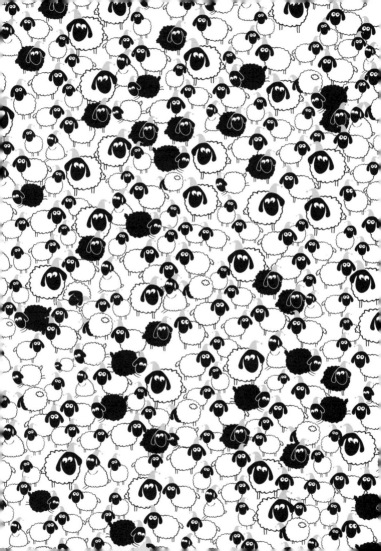

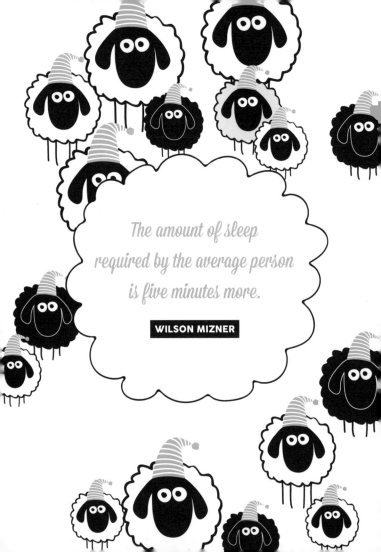

The amount of sleep
required by the average person
is five minutes more.

WILSON MIZNER

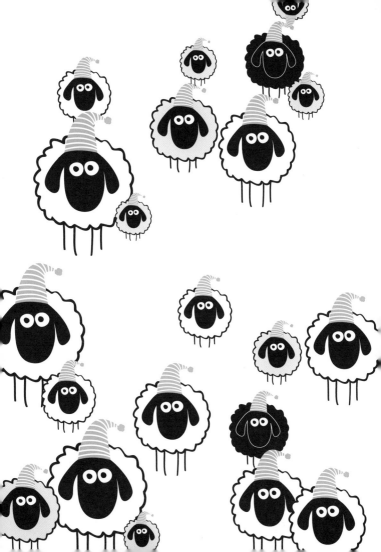

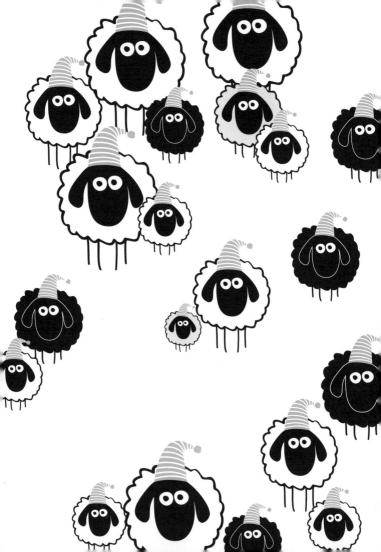

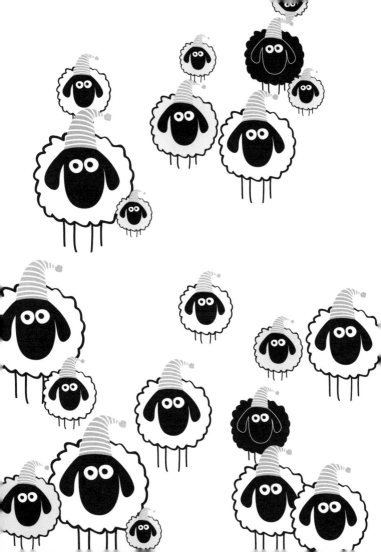

FIND THE PAIR

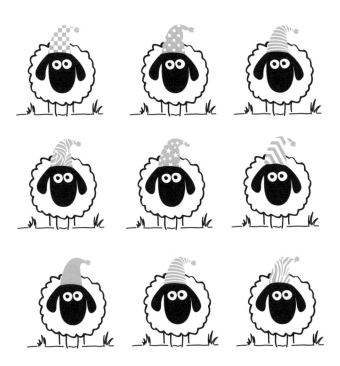

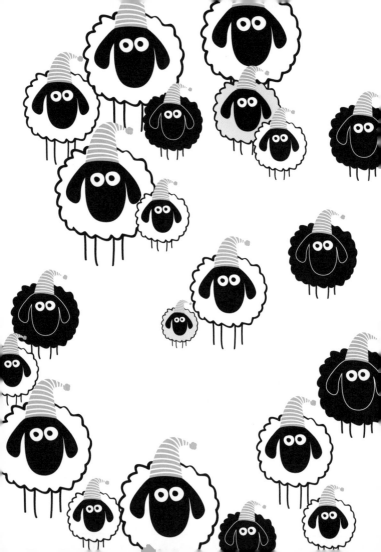

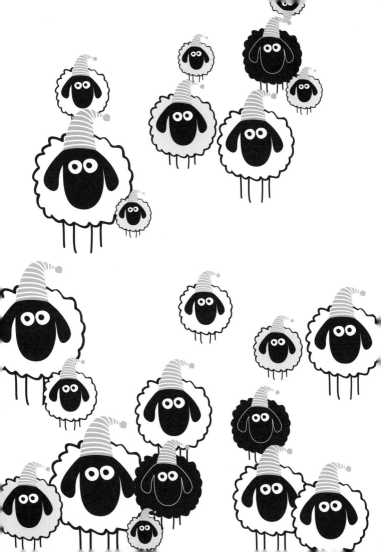

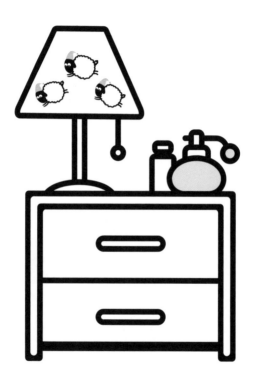

HAVE GENTLE LIGHTING
IN YOUR BEDROOM TO HELP
EASE THE TRANSITION
FROM DAY TO NIGHT.
THE SOFTER LIGHT WILL
HELP SIGNAL TO YOUR BODY
THAT IT'S TIME TO SLEEP.

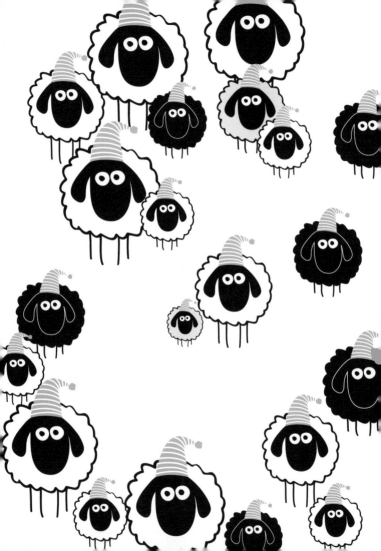

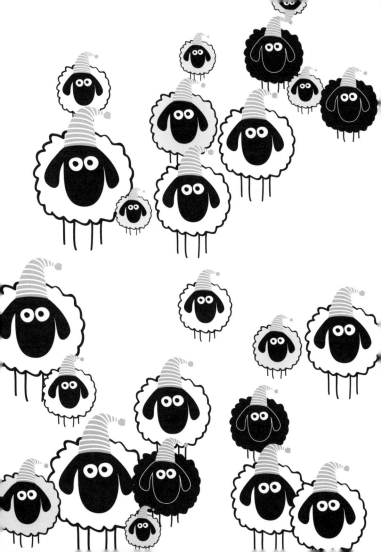

FIND THE PAIR

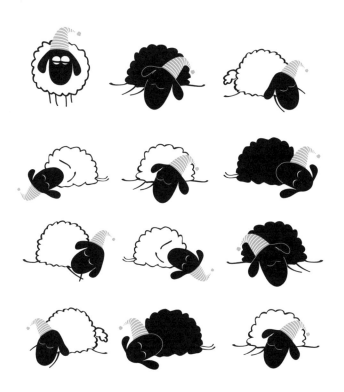

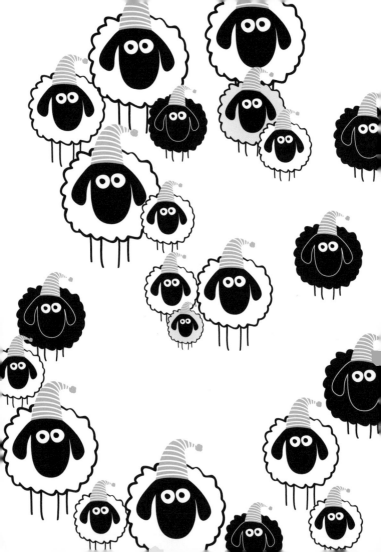

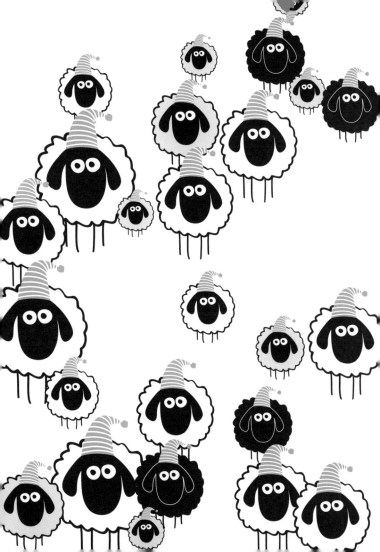

GUIDE KIP TO THE PILLOW

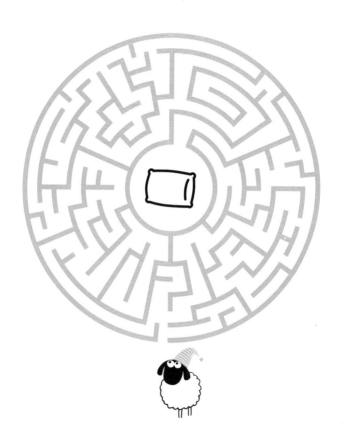

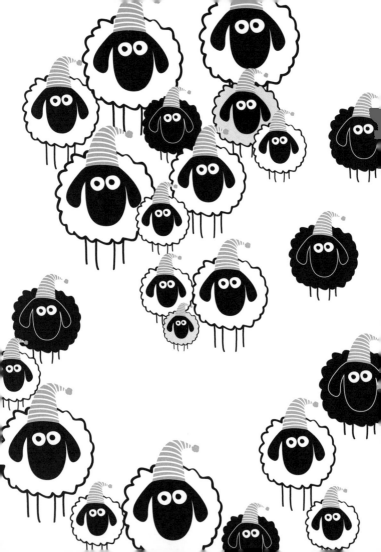

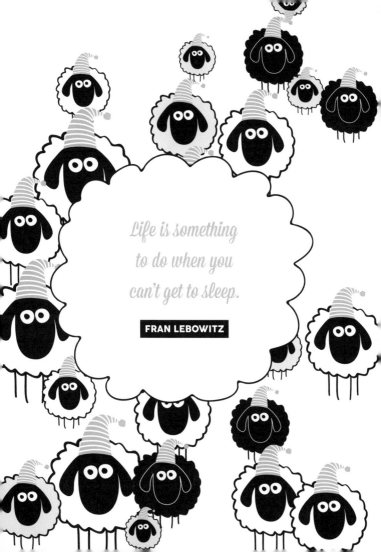

Life is something
to do when you
can't get to sleep.

FRAN LEBOWITZ

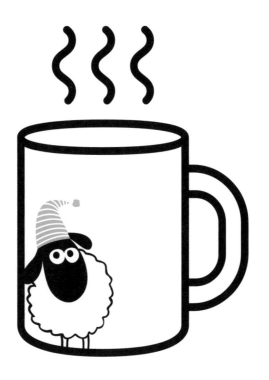

Enjoy a warm drink before you go to bed, such as fruit tea, herbal tea, or a cup of warm milk, to soothe you into sleep.

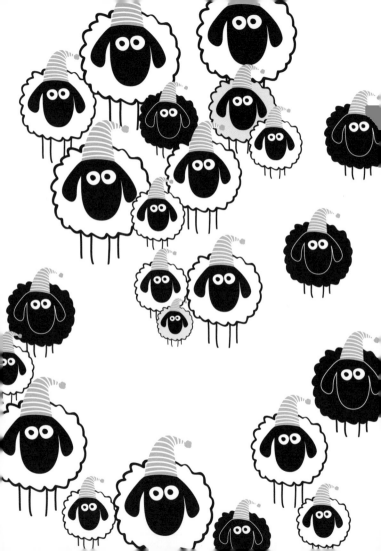

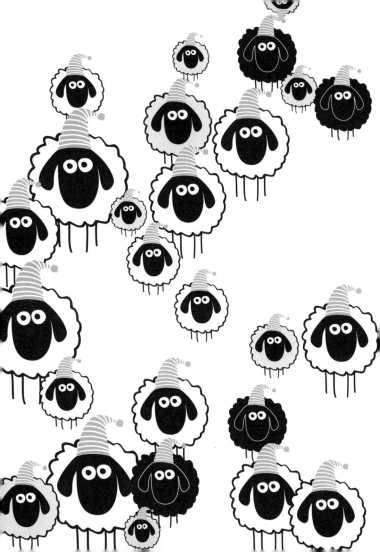

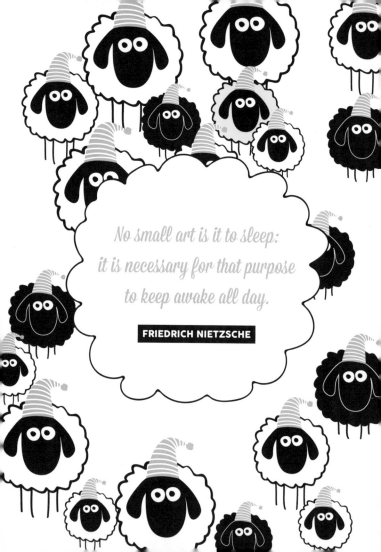

No small art is it to sleep:
it is necessary for that purpose
to keep awake all day.

FRIEDRICH NIETZSCHE

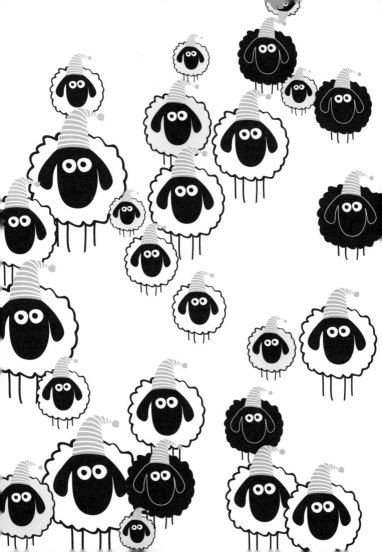

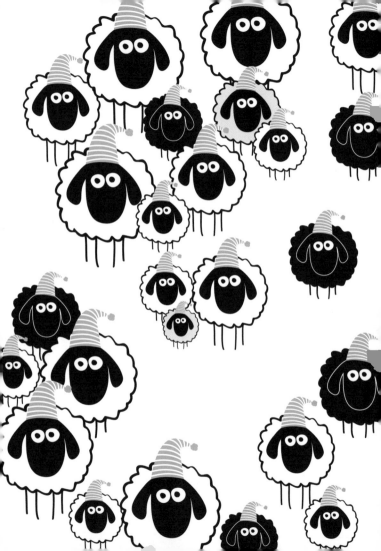

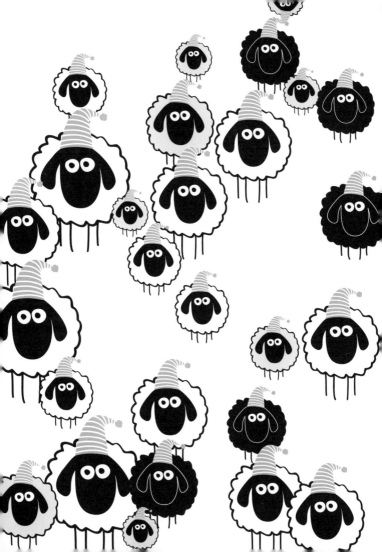

GUIDE KIP TO THE PILLOW

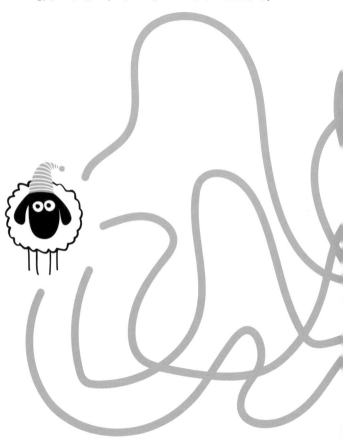

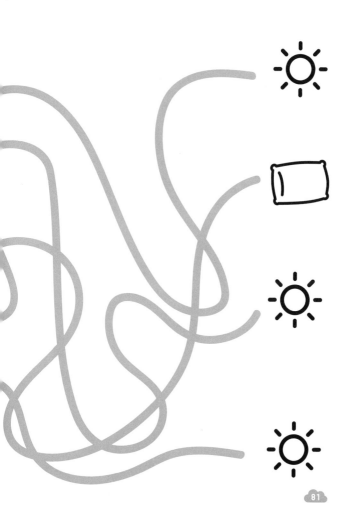

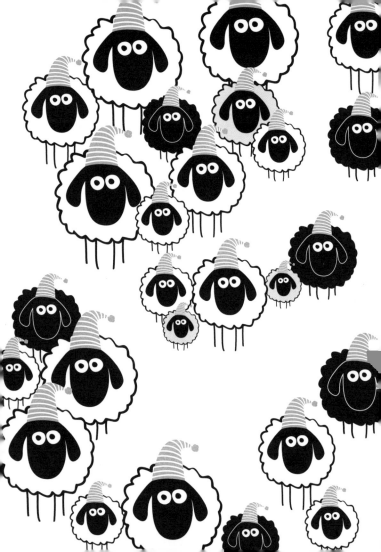

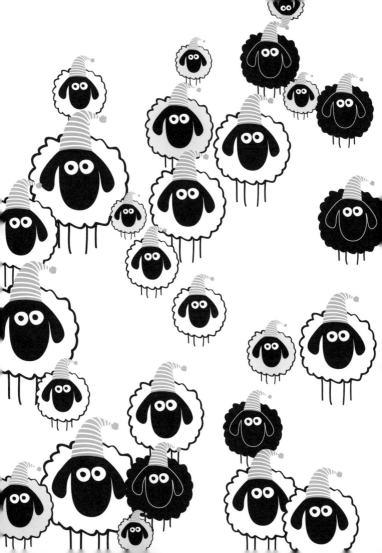

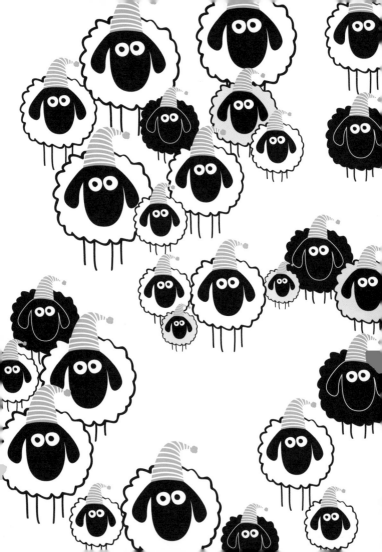

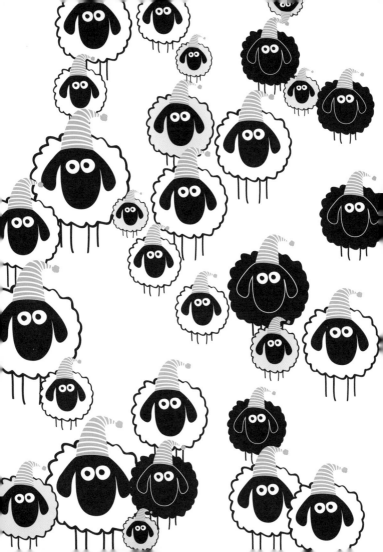

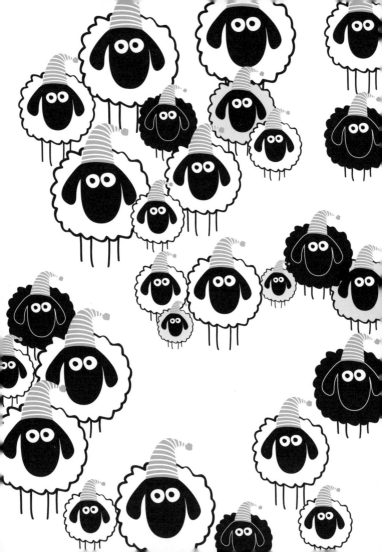

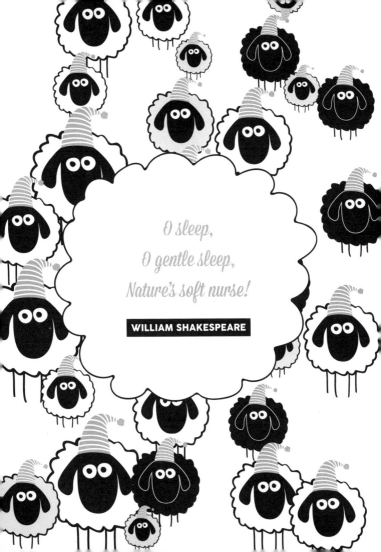

O sleep,
O gentle sleep,
Nature's soft nurse!

WILLIAM SHAKESPEARE

GUIDE KIP TO THE PILLOW

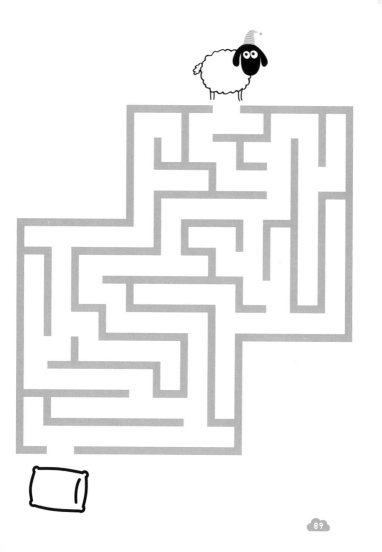

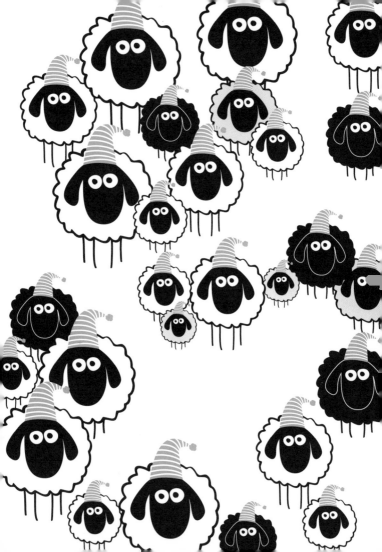

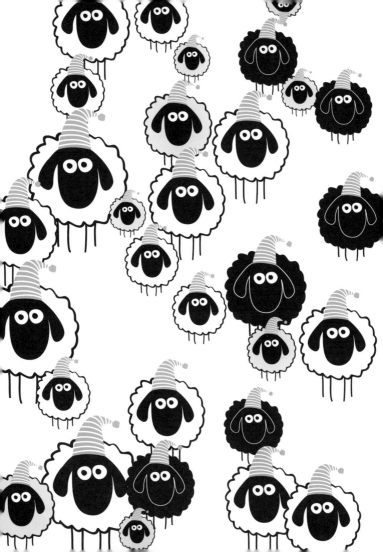

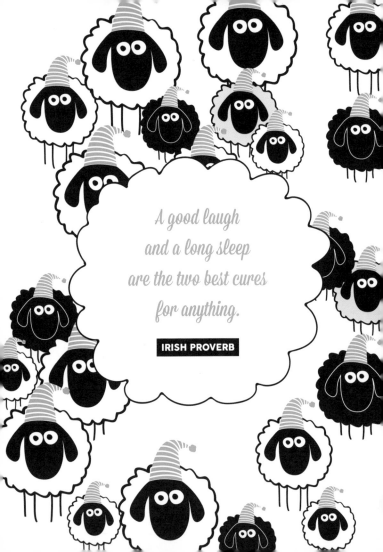

A good laugh
and a long sleep
are the two best cures
for anything.

IRISH PROVERB

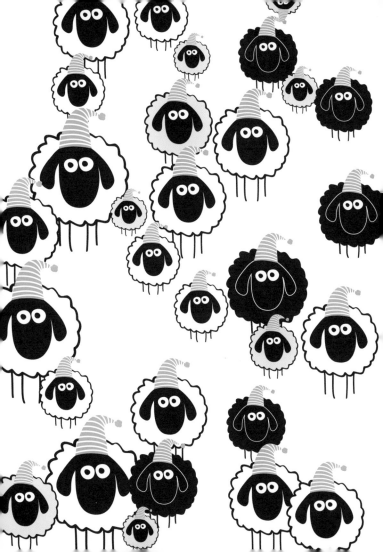

SPOT THE FIVE DIFFERENCES

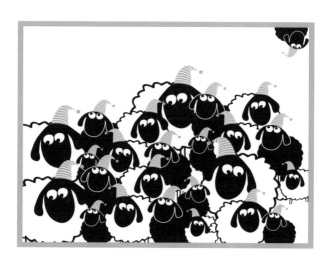

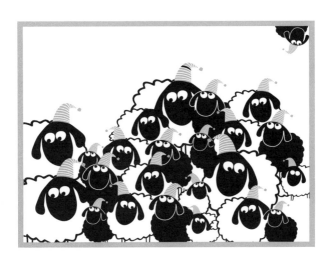

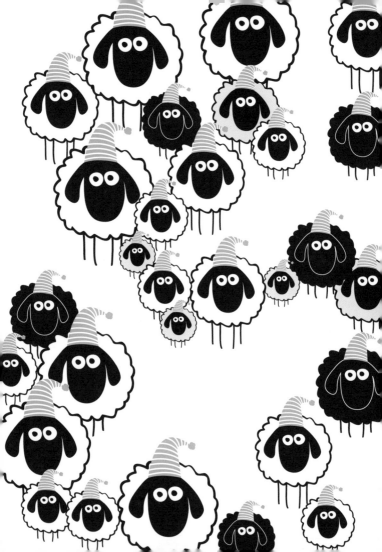

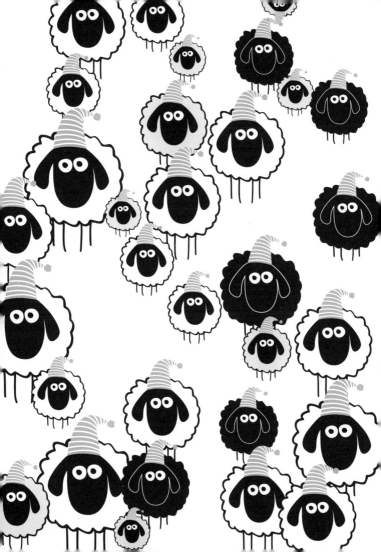

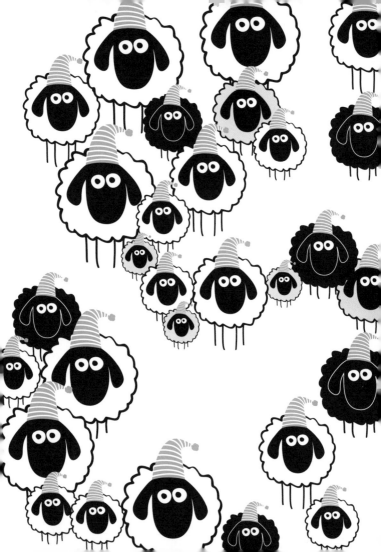

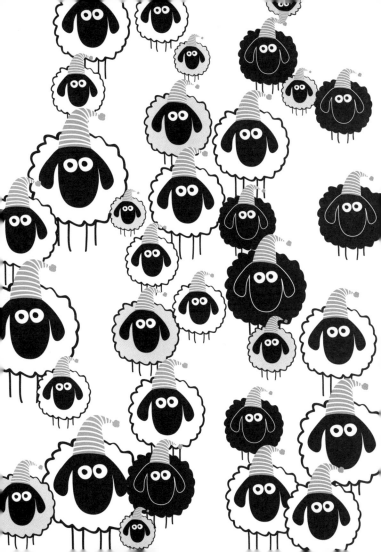

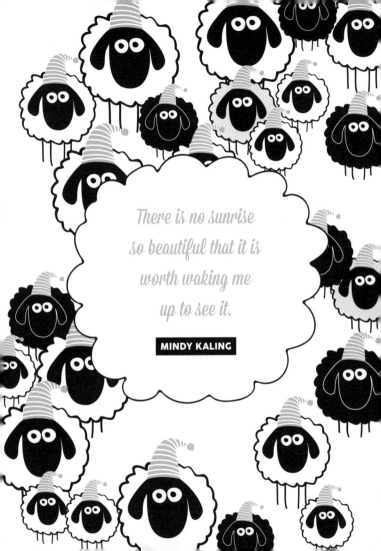

There is no sunrise so beautiful that it is worth waking me up to see it.

MINDY KALING

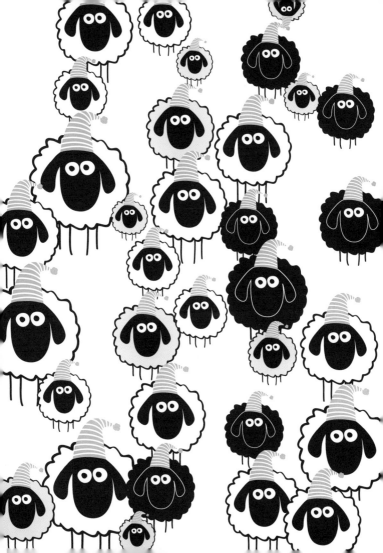

Find "Calm"

m	c	a	c	a	m	a	c
c	m	a	m	l	c	a	c
a	l	m	l	c	m	m	a
l	a	c	a	l	a	l	m
a	m	a	m	c	l	a	l
m	l	a	l	m	a	c	c
l	a	l	m	l	m	a	l
a	m	c	a	c	a	m	a

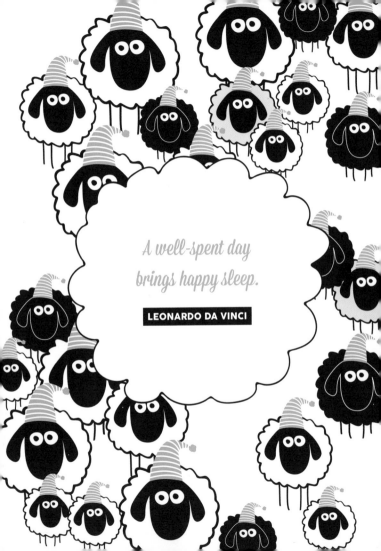

A well-spent day
brings happy sleep.

LEONARDO DA VINCI

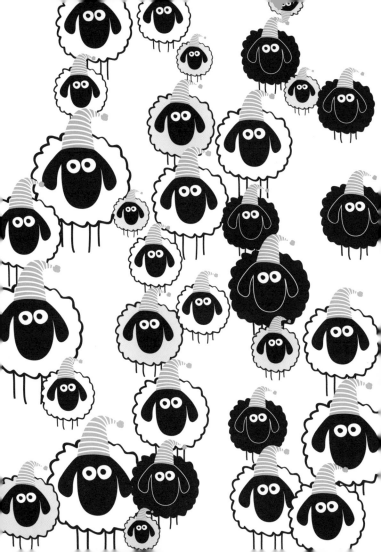

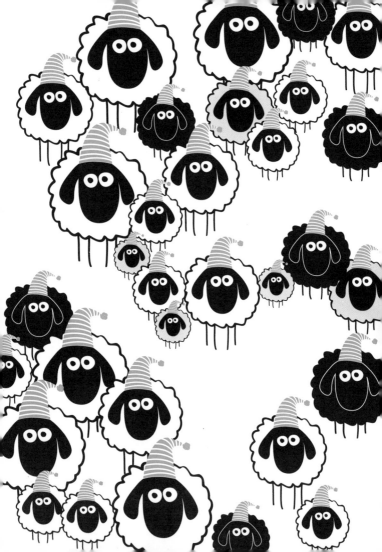

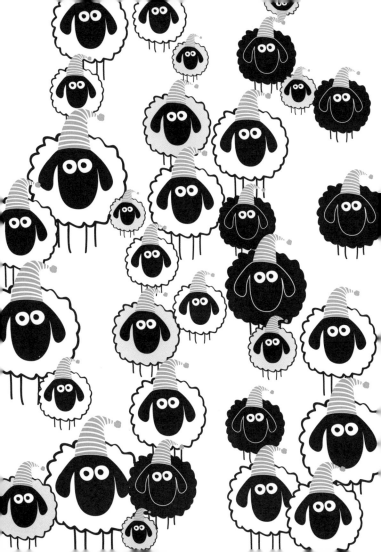

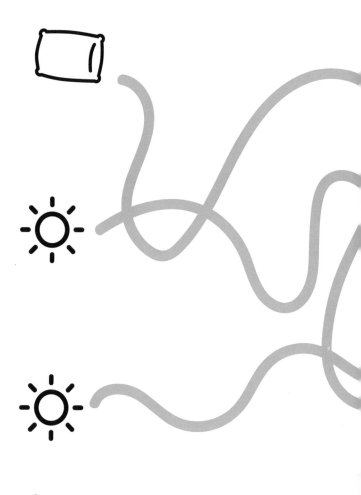

GUIDE KIP TO THE PILLOW

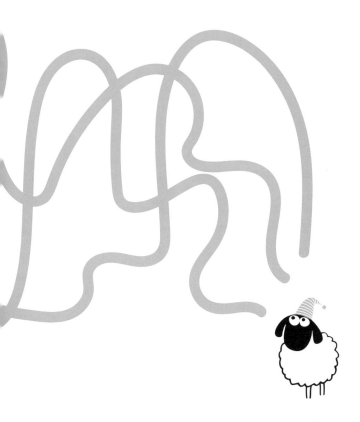

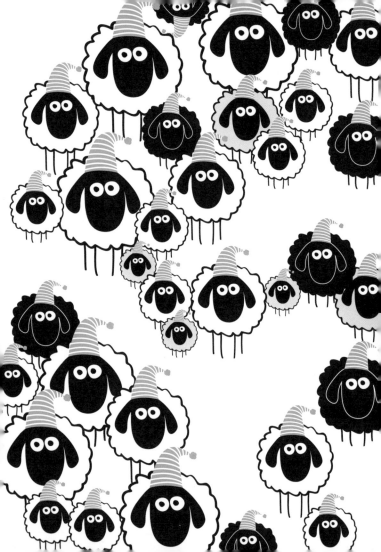

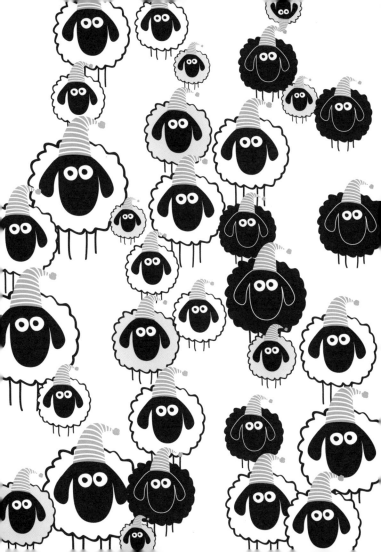

FIND THE PILLOW

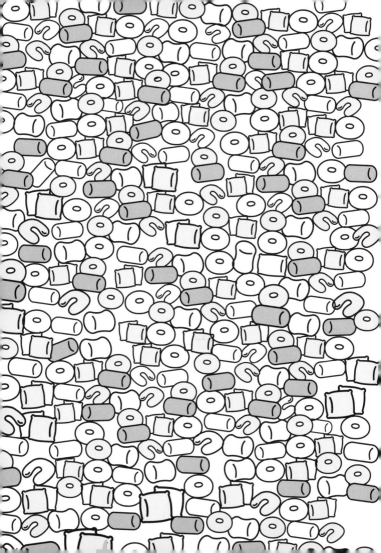

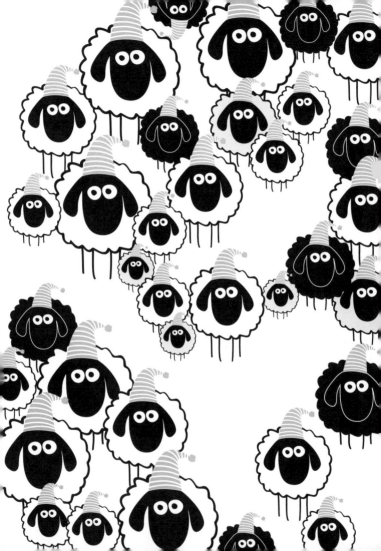

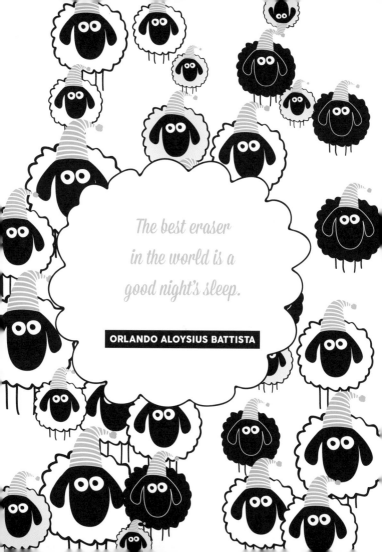

The best eraser
in the world is a
good night's sleep.

ORLANDO ALOYSIUS BATTISTA

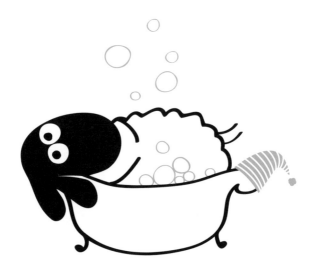

A soothing bath is a wonderful way to relax your mind and body before bed. Add your favorite bubbles or essential oils to make it extra special.

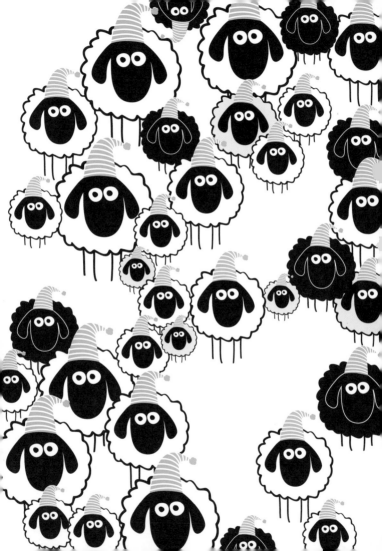

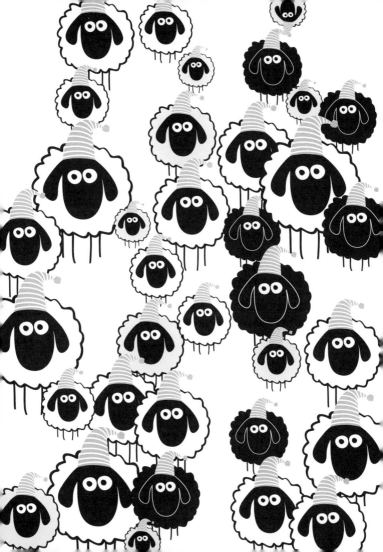

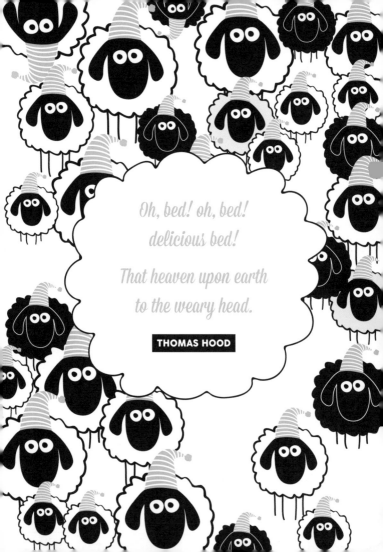

Oh, bed! oh, bed!
delicious bed!

That heaven upon earth
to the weary head.

THOMAS HOOD

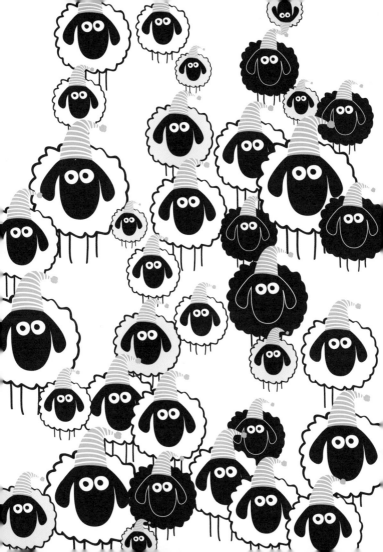

Help Kip
catch some Zzzs

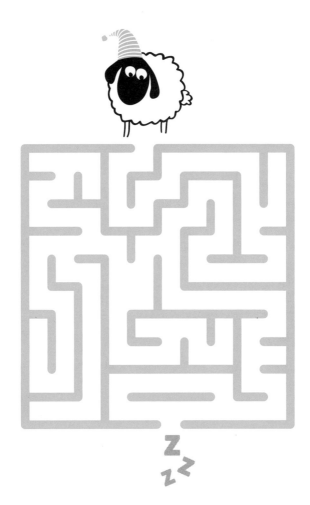

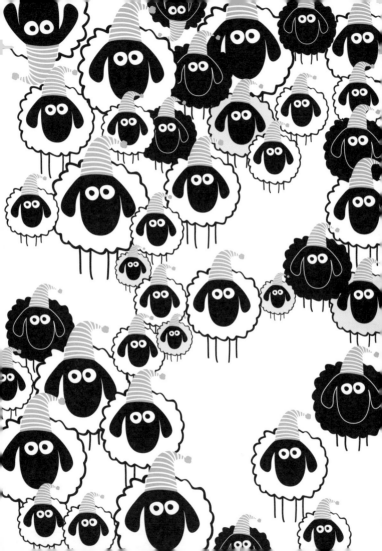

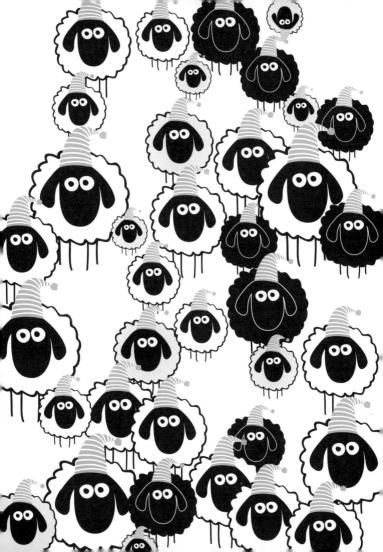

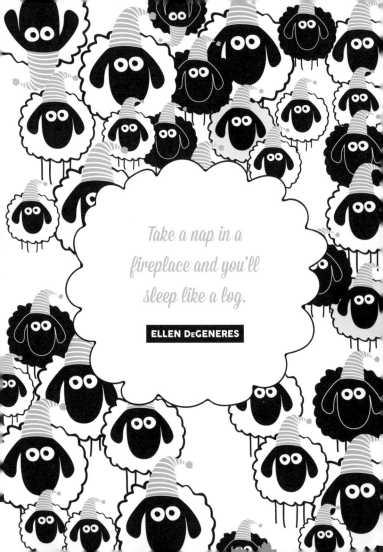

Take a nap in a fireplace and you'll sleep like a log.

ELLEN DeGENERES

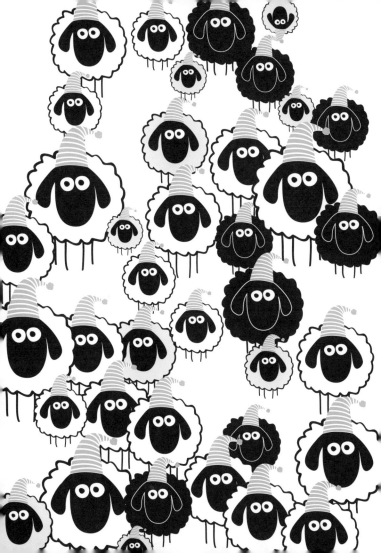

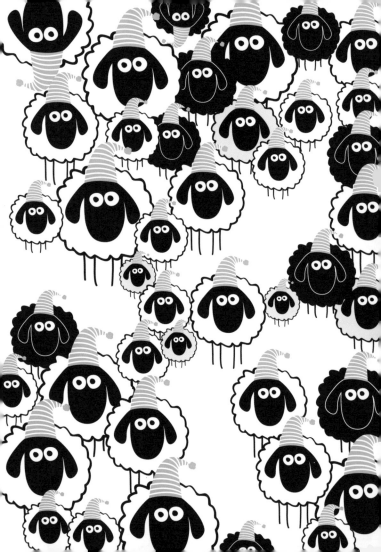

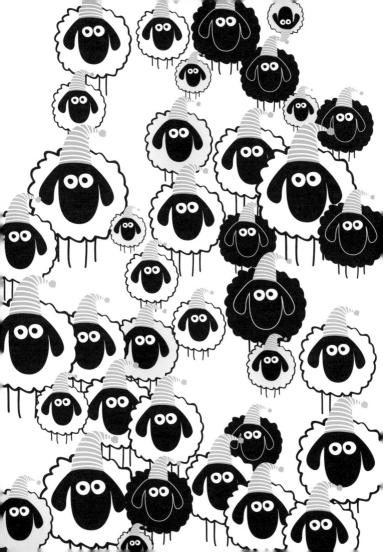

GUIDE KIP TO THE PILLOW

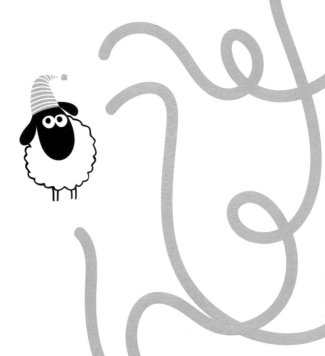

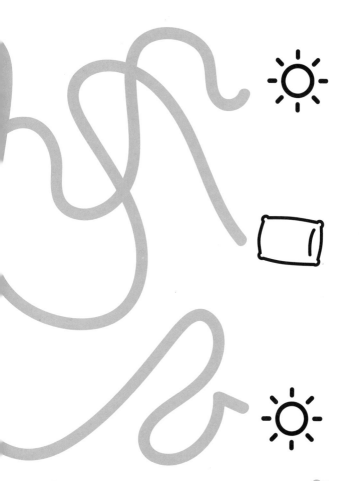

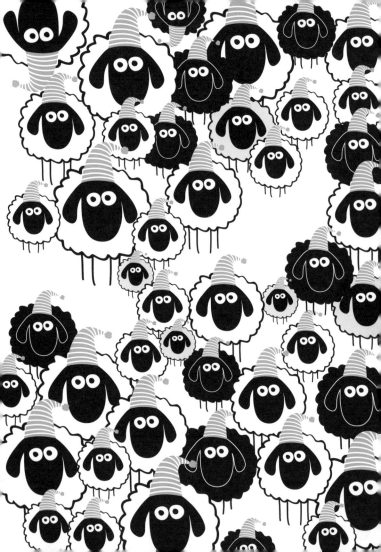

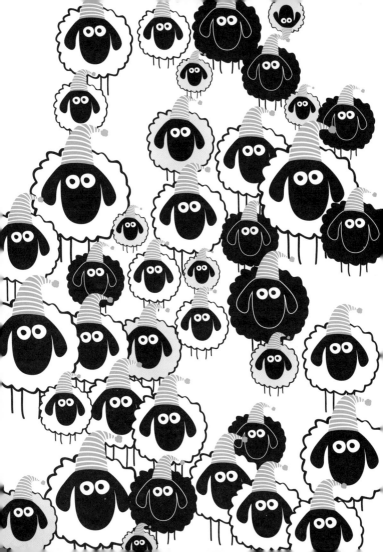

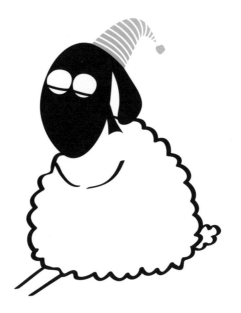

Sit anywhere you feel comfortable and close your eyes. Breathe in slowly through your nose until your lungs are full. Hold for four slow counts, then exhale slowly. Repeat until you are feeling calm.

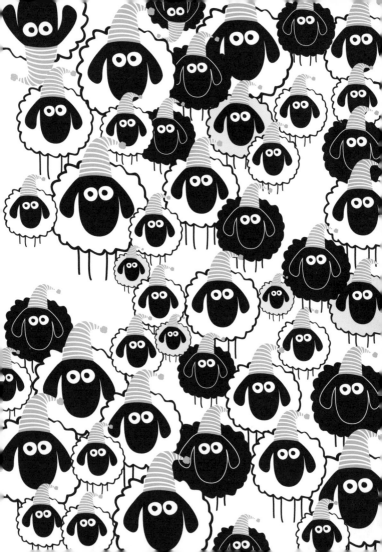

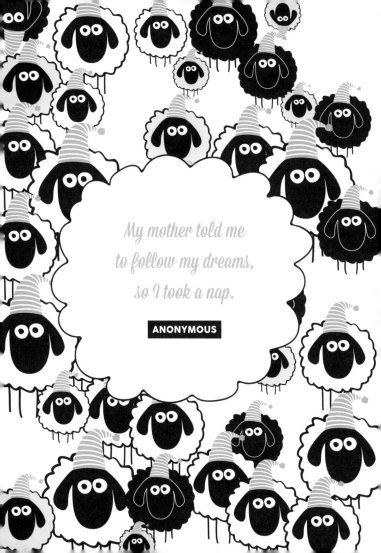

My mother told me
to follow my dreams,
so I took a nap.

ANONYMOUS

FIND THE PAIR

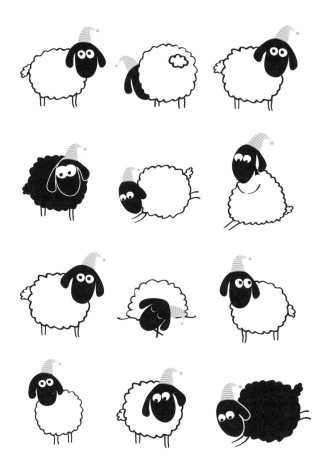

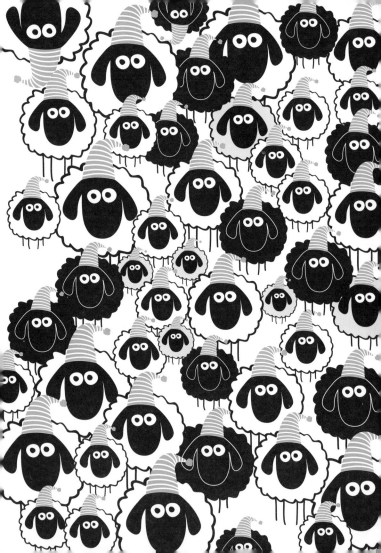

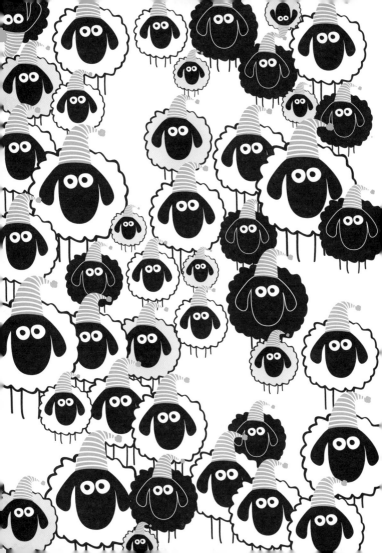

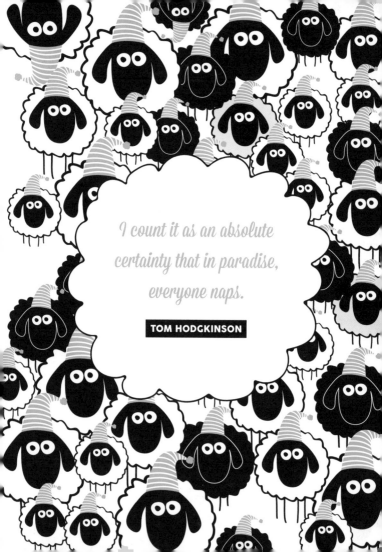

I count it as an absolute certainty that in paradise, everyone naps.

TOM HODGKINSON

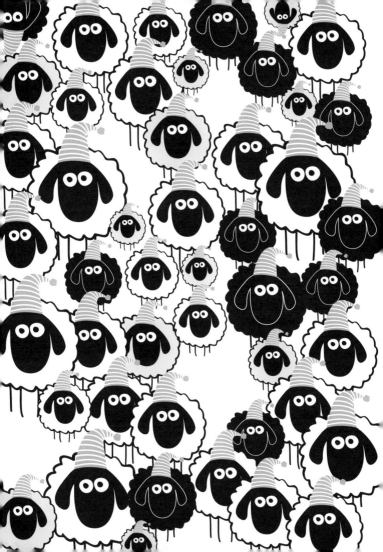

Complete the word search

bedtime

sleep

shut-eye

relax

slumber

forty winks

s	k	n	i	w	y	t	r	o	f	p	t
l	k	j	h	g	f	d	s	e	t	r	s
p	o	u	y	u	t	s	l	e	e	p	l
a	e	n	h	u	r	h	v	q	t	s	a
t	f	m	o	f	c	u	x	s	s	q	v
m	w	e	i	r	u	t	k	n	l	m	c
h	f	l	n	t	f	e	g	y	u	p	z
q	u	f	v	c	d	y	e	w	m	a	s
l	t	r	e	s	x	e	u	q	b	z	w
p	q	y	r	d	v	b	b	o	e	j	u
r	e	l	a	x	q	k	s	n	r	o	p
c	h	v	e	w	i	h	v	l	m	u	x

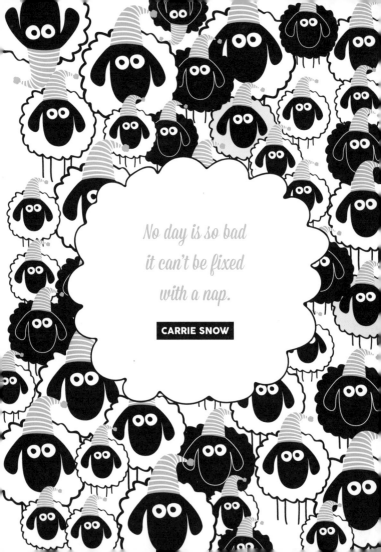

No day is so bad it can't be fixed with a nap.

CARRIE SNOW

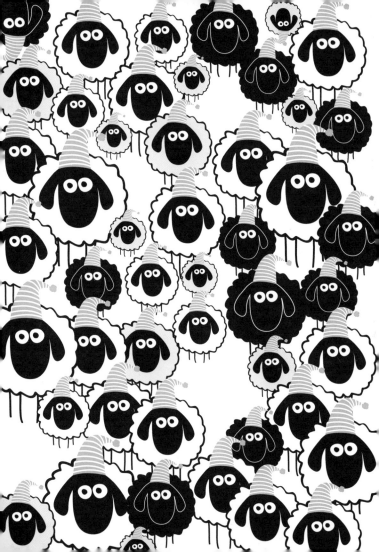

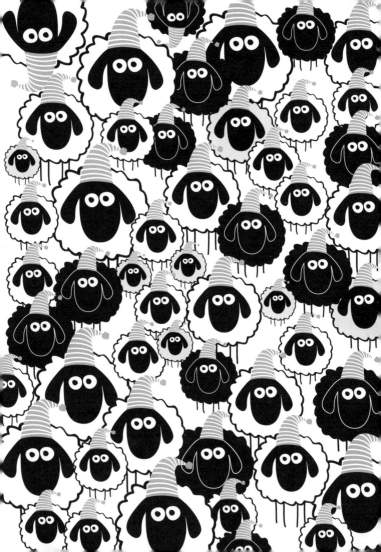

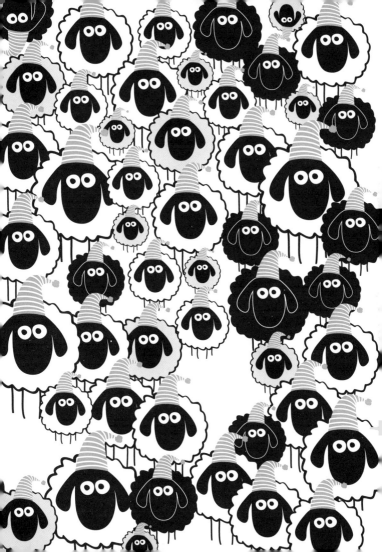

Spot the five differences

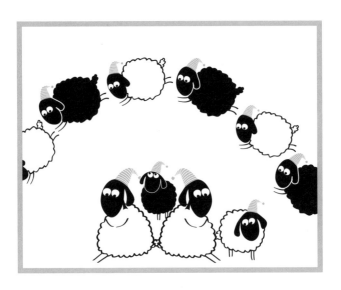

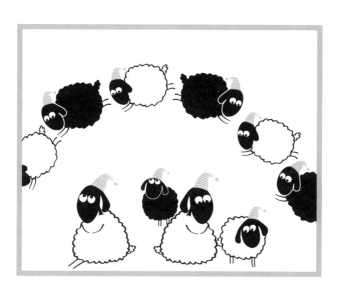

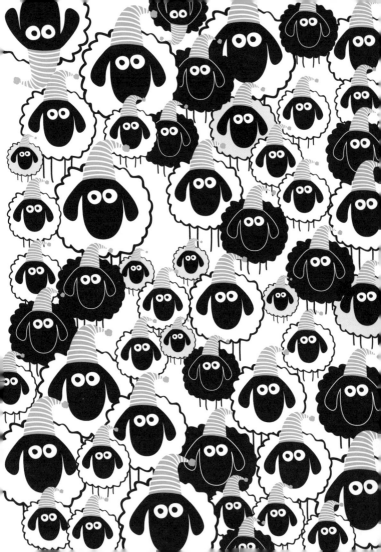

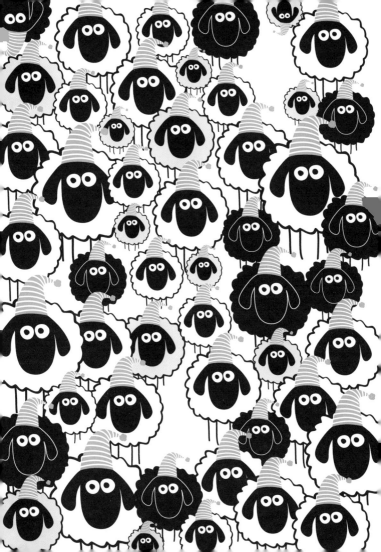

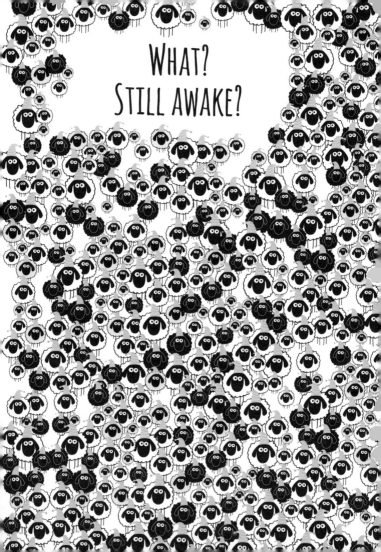

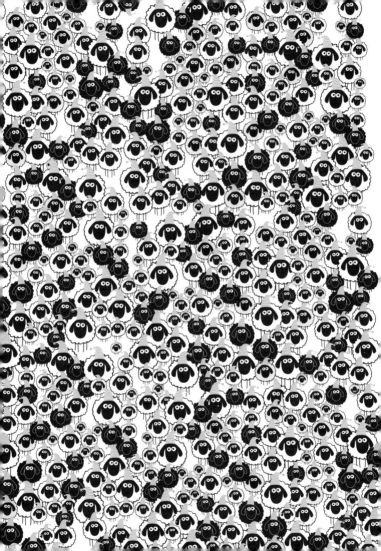

SWEET DREAMS

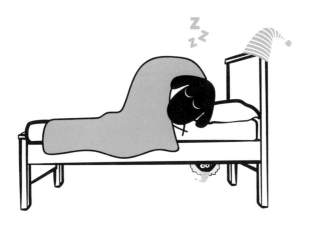

ANSWERS

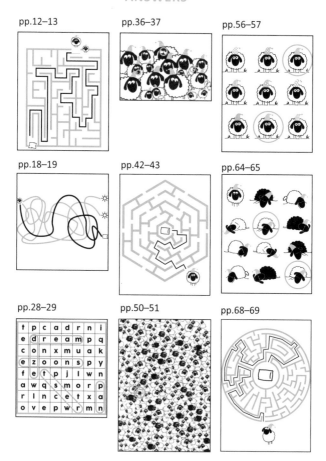

pp.12–13

pp.36–37

pp.56–57

pp.18–19

pp.42–43

pp.64–65

pp.28–29

pp.50–51

pp.68–69

pp.80–81

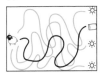

pp.108–109

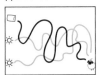

pp.130–131

pp.88–89

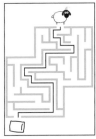

pp.112–113

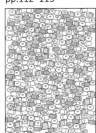

pp.138–139

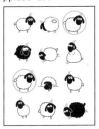

pp.94–95

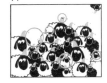

pp.122–123

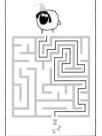

pp.144–145

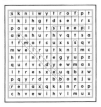

pp.102–103

m	c	a	c	a	m	a	c
c	m	a	m	l	c	a	c
a	l	m	l	c	m	m	a
l	a	c	a	l	a	l	m
a	m	a	m	c	l	a	l
m	l	a	l	m	a	c	c
l	a	l	m	l	m	a	l
a	m	c	a	c	a	m	a

pp.150–151

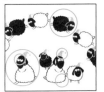

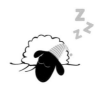

IMAGE CREDITS